PMS: A Guy's Roadmap
(In case you won't ask for directions.)

PMS: A Guy's Roadmap
(In case you won't ask for directions.)

The secrets to living with a lady's cycle

Kay Christianson

Writer's Showcase
San Jose New York Lincoln Shanghai

PMS: A Guy's Roadmap (In case you won't ask for directions.)
The secrets to living with a lady's cycle

Writer's Showcase
an imprint of iUniverse.com, Inc.

For information address:
iUniverse.com, Inc.
5220 S 16th, Ste. 200
Lincoln, NE 68512
www.iuniverse.com

There were no animals harmed in the making of this book.
But some were nervous.

ISBN: 0-595-15882-X

Printed in the United States of America

To Mom, the classiest lady I've ever known.
(You could never even discern her cycle.)

Epigraph

"Just remember, we're all in this alone." Lily Tomlin.

"Never eat more than you can lift." Miss Piggy

Contents

List of Tables

The Politically-Correct Preface

As a PMS guidebook, let me begin by saying this book features pages and pages of scientific data, which, though clinically proven, is in no way meant to be taken, well, seriously. Therefore, don't try to use this as an admission that women are somehow ineffective professionally, politically or in any other way, because of a physical circumstance. Our worst days are some of our most productive. Our PMS eccentricities often lead to cleaner homes, more organized businesses, and better performance by your local Senator.

The following pages have been treated with a chemical substance similar to that which preserves pork rinds, and which will chemically react with the skin pH of anyone who has no sense of humor. And said reader's lips will fall off. This however, usually takes a month, or as much time as it takes to write letters of feminine protest to a publisher.

Acknowledgements

Special thanks to Alice, Virgil, Kellie, Kurt, Sue, Deb and everyone forced to proofread various chapters. I really wasn't interested in typos…just how hard you laughed while you looked for them. Thank goodness you did. And added thanks to my sister, for being the first person I really credit for teaching me that just about everything is funny.

The Introduction

Yes, you may be thinking, "Kay, the important part of the book hasn't started? Another preface, introduction, forward thingy? To the untrained eye, it may appear there are many issues to be covered, though the procrastinator instantly recognizes his own kind. No, seriously, this *is* the important part of the book. The rest is just fodder to fill enough pages to make it commercially viable, which the commercially astute also recognize.

In any case, I for one, have PMS right now, which means, of course, there is a bag of fries to the left of me and what's left of a hot-fudge sundae on my right. It seemed only appropriate that I write the book's introduction under these conditions, though certainly not the whole book, as PMS is only a brief, fleeting, and temporary condition. It's also one that can yield great periods of intense productivity for a woman. So read on. I'm done. There. That took 4 seconds.

For all you lost and confused males out there, this book attempts to clarify…to reveal female mysteries…and to make it easier for you to watch the Superbowl unencumbered.

When it comes to things menstrual, men are uncomfortable hearing about the subject from their women. Or perhaps, the only time they share information is in the "thick of the battle" in which case, the only discernable answer these men get is, "It's filthy in here, get me some potato chips!"

Men are equally uncomfortable *talking* about it, as they are most subjects. Therefore, the topic may only be touched upon during some male-bonding event, like watching basketball playoffs, the discourse sounding something like this: "Shoot! Shoot!!! Yeah. So, Andrea out shopping? Yeah. Does she get weird at that time?…Shoot!! Don't get it, man. Yeah. Pass the pretzels."

This ultimately produces nothing more than a grunt, deep belch, and a look of male-bonded contentment. But, it leaves the participants with no more understanding of the subject than they had in the fifth grade, (fresh from that weird health class they had to bring a special permission slip to go to).

So, for all you males who are never sure…who are at a loss for what to do every 28 days…who would prefer to peruse the answers via the complete anonymity of the printed word. Or for those who need to buy their brother-in-law a fairly inexpensive birthday gift quickly, this book is for you. And for the women who live with you.

Chapter 1

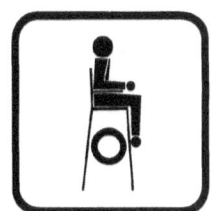

Knowing...when she doesn't

Gentlemen, living with a woman who experiences PMS bears heavy responsibility, not unlike the military responsibility of avoiding the red button during nuclear crisis.

You see, the difficulty lies in the fact that PMS creeps up on a woman. It's camouflaged. Like an evil little parasite that sucks the life and vibrance from its victim, depositing a venom which sucks the life force drop by drop from its hapless host...oh. I digress. The point is, no matter how accurate her "calendar," the PMS schedule can vary. One month, it's five days before detonation, the next, it's two. And because it varies and progressively intensifies, your lady may not always recognize the onslaught until the mushroom cloud is dissipating. That's why it's critical that you can. *Your* being able to identify the condition in that first day or so is critical to making the most of the next few.

(Insert helpful male-oriented reference here:)

It's sort of like, in basketball, being able to recognize when your team's forward has a knee injury that's gonna get worse, even when the guy insists on playing, so that you have time to counter-bet the serious chunk of change you had riding on these playoffs...Get it? There's value in figuring this stuff out.

Knowing how to accurately "diagnose" the condition, if you will, is a potent tool. (Did you like how I used the phrase "Potent tool?" This book could give you a potent tool. Tell your friends.) Properly identifying PMS is crucial to making the most of it.

"But how?" You ask. "I have a foggy notion that she gets a little cranky sometimes…as do we all. She gets a hankering for some odd food…as do we all. There are even times in which she *wants* to clean. But what's the difference between these occurrences and true PMS?" It's the discerning and wise, nay, potent man who can distinguish between a "bad day" and full force PMS. So, to assist you until you become adept at this, I've included this handy quiz:

A QUIZ: Are You Dealing With PMS?

Consider the following common circumstances, and compare your lady's typical responses with those in this scientific chart…

IRRITATING CIRCUMSTANCE:	JUST A BAD DAY:	PMS:
•She whistles off to the laundry room and suddenly discovers the wash load is too large to fit in the machine...	"Why don't *you* do the stupid wash this week anyway!"	Many words are indiscernible between sobs, but you'd swear her tirade had something to do with the children in Peru not having enough clothes...
•You forget to feed the dog...	A can of Alpo is set on your dinner plate.	Divorce papers are promptly filed.
• She is late for a client meeting at the office...	Snaps at the receptionist when queried about her arrival.	Upon arrival to the meeting, she exhibits an unusual altering of make-up and accessories. For example, a corn dog stick protrudes from her pocket, and she sports a chocolate puddin' mustache.
• You stroll in the door and say, "hello"...	"And what's *that* supposed to mean?"	She wears rubber gloves and shakes a can of Comet in your general direction proclaiming, "*This place is a pig-stye, and if you think she's going to sit in the midst of it for even one minute, you're got another thing coming.*" You escort her through theatre doors by distracting her with a large popcorn (extra butter). The show's about to start.
• She runs out of gas...	She recounts a story to you incorporating expletives the likes of which you haven't heard since visiting uncle Ned in the Turret's syndrome ward of the state hospital.	She's overly-concerned with whether this outfit makes her look "hippy". She's speaking of the orange jail-issue coveralls she's sporting after hijacking a Chevron gas truck with nothing but her bare hands and "The Club" from her steering wheel.
• You go to rent a movie...	She insists on "Thelma & Louise"	It's a toss-up between "The Bridges of Madison County," "Terms of Endearment" and "Old Yeller".

** **WARNING**: If too many days are spent in column 2 above, what's wrong with you? Get outta there. Column 3 is much more normal.

Compare your lady's behaviors with these and test your diagnostic skills. Of course, she probably exhibits far more than 5 behaviors in life.

So, the author recognizes that this chart is a little brief, but, you should be getting the idea.

I recognize you may now have questions arising, so I will attempt to brush them aside here.

"Is there something I can give her to make it go away?"
A week's stay at a health spa should do the trick.

Clearly the only way to rid yourself of the problem is to rid yourself of her for a few days, and if this is not economically feasible, return half the shoes she bought last month, and that should help.

"Is there something she can take to help?"
A week off. See the previous question.

"Do all the symptoms come together?"
Often. If your lady is exhibiting signs of emotional upheaval, insatiable appetite, sexual yearnings for Mr. Clean, and a swelling stomach, (and she's not a Klingon), she definitely is experiencing PMS.

"What about menopause?"
That's the subject of another book. Which I'll write in about 18 years.

"Do men experience sympathetic PMS disorders?"
Yes. Many scientific journals describe this phenomenon as, "the irrepressible urge to go bowling with the guys, play some ball with the guys, and/or, but not limited to, the need to leave and play guitars with the guys."

"How do you determine the progression and seriousness of the condition?"

The previous method of measurement, "hps" or, "hormones per second" has since been proved inaccurate and impractical, due to the difficulty in implementation for the average non-micro-biologist, let alone you. Today, PMS severity is commonly measured in, "tpm's" or tears per minute. If her tpm count has escalated beyond say, the quantity of the water-tower capacity of a small town in Arkansas, you've probably got an advanced case on your hands.

"How do I know when it's ended?"

When it seems to be escalating. (Get a calendar and count back 3 weeks. There's the ending date, which you obviously missed. Pay more attention next time.) This would likely mean you missed the end of the last cycle by 4 weeks and we're starting over.

"What do I do when I know she's got PMS, but she screams she doesn't (while cleaning the hall closet for the third time?)"

Agree with her. It turns out many women don't recognize the early signs of PMS, which coincidentally, are often confused with minor felonies, so the unnoticeability is understandable.

"When does she recognize and admit its effects?"

When she sees them in her grandchildren.

"Couldn't she be using the PMS thing as an excuse for just a short temper, especially when I calculate it's probably the *middle* of her cycle?"

Don't be an idiot. Haven't you ever heard of repressed memory?

"What about when she notices she has PMS and it calms her down, but if *I* mention it, she divorces me?"

How dare you.

Of course, maybe it's you.

A great many of women's frustrations in the world are, in a word, men. So it's important to do some self-examination, which I will gently guide you through here. Are the mood swings chemical, or are you just a pompous-idiot-of-a-self-indulgent-creep-without-a-thought-for-another-human-but-yourself? (A condition which could, if left untreated, mimic in a reactionary fashion, the symptoms of PMS in your lady.)

Let's find out.

QUIZ: PMS—Or, You're a Jerk?

Are your lady's typical responses to you PMS-oriented, or do you just deserve them?

IRRITATING CIRCUMSTANCE:	PMS...	JERK...
• She suddenly snaps and says she's moving out because of the mess you make. —She's speaking after the 3rd visit from the health department... — She's speaking after her third Ding Dong...	.......√	.......√
• Your shaving goo lining the sink has accumulated to such proportion she's threatening to clean your closet again. When compiled, it does seem to rival, in appearance, Cousin It...		.......√
• She hits the roof when she sees you press a wadded-up tube sock against your nose to see if just couldn't be worn one more time...		.......√
• There is a plethora of empty beer bottles, "strewn all over the kitchen", making her nauseous. The total is rapidly climbing to, say, two...	.......√	
• She weeps uncontrollably because the dirty pans you left in the sink remind her of Dr. Zivago...	.......√	
• "You let out another stinker like" that and she's chucking your World Series baseball in the nearest dishwasher. — She realizes you didn't fart, she did ...but the threat still stands...	.......√	.......√
• She refuses to let you go to the lake, let alone, join you. You're wearing socks and a Speedo.	......√	.......√
• "You are clearly the most thoughtless bum on earth." You forgot the extra salt for the Dino-fries.	.......√	
• Your lady announces to the entire restaurant that you fart in your sleep. Repeatedly. (Her announcement, that is.) You're there on a date with her cousin.	......√	.......√

Remember too, that women, including your beloved, are often the hapless victims of the onslaught, which, in English, means it's never our fault. Could it be yours?

Without the skill for identifying PMS, men are left orchestrating a beautiful tap dance in which they spin round and round the floor, in a graceful whirl, and land a breathless and confused heap for the next 25 days or so. But with this skill, you're left in a confused heap for about 2 fewer days.

Congratulations. You finished the first chapter with no more answers than you had when you began. Relax. The answers come later. Now you know you have to recognize the signs when she doesn't, but you don't know how. If we've gotten you that far, my work here is done.

Chapter 2

The Cycle Is Like A Football Game

The author has come to realize that many men do not seem to comprehend the "menstrual cycle" in terms of its actual "schedule," as well as they comprehend say, the complex rules of football. "When is PMS? When is ovulation? When does one phenomenon start and another end, and the cycle repeat itself?"

This fact is surprising, considering this very gender created a game which, at face value, centers around carrying a lemon drop-shaped pig skin across a field for 100 yards, while the opposing team knocks you over along the way. This concept sounds simple, yet men infused this basic structure with "rules and regulations" so confounding the average nuclear physicist would spend their time playing chopsticks if splitting an atom were so complex. Which probably explains why nuclear physicists don't play football, but I digress.

No, the simple concept of football involves complex details, such as • a kick off, • 7 point-scoring, but not always because sometimes it's one or two, • legal slamming and head-butting, • illegal slamming and headbutting, • off-sides for attempting to slam and head-but too early, • angry scowls from coaches for attempting to slam and head-butt too late, • lots of padding to protect players bodies from the detriments of slamming and headbutting because clearly slamming

and head-butting is bad for you, that's why we built a game around it, •
a first-down which must be proceeded by three more or else nothing's
gone down, • turn-overs which have nothing to do with apples, • arm-
waving referees recruited from flight decks of aircraft carriers but without their flashlights, • sticks and flags which measure within inches the
additional length a ball has fallen beyond the bloody mass which previously was #42's outstretched right arm, • over-time • half-time in which
women with slightly less padding in their bras than the players, scamper
about the field amidst marching bands who we wish to slam and head-
butt as they spell out clever things like USC! where the tuba provides
the dot to the exclamation point. This my friends, is all surprisingly
similar to what we women like to call "the menstruation game".

Hence, the football game analogy.

Men, rest assured. If you can comprehend football, we'll get you to
grasp your lady's physical schedules. The football game analogy goes
something like this…

Imagine a 30-day football game that never stops repeating itself. As
soon as the game is over…a new one starts right up.

Now, before you fall over in an orgasmic-pleasure-fit, think of it as a
30-day football game, and try to grasp some definitions.

Menstruation is like the kick-off…

Day One. Aunt Flo has taken her seat on the fifty-yard line. The game
is underway.

Each of the first four *days* or first four *plays* is like a Down…

On average, you need at least 4 downs before Auntie leaves the field
and goes back to the locker room to wait for the start of the next game.
(She's kind of like a kicker)

Now, after 4 downs… the game is in full swing. Everyone's pretty
happy. Enthusiasm throughout the stadium is running high, but nobody's

in the clinch. There's time to get a beer. Everyone sitting near you is in a pretty good mood…but half time is approaching…and half time counts.

Halftime = Ovulation.

As day 14 of this month-long game approaches, half-time preparations begin. Remember when you had the crush on that cheerleader in school? She was gonna come out at half time and do a really bad dance in a really short skirt to some old song by "Journey"? And how did that short skirt make you feel? Exactly. Half time approaches and your lady's getting horny.

That's because nature's drive to procreate has a built-in system which hormonally over-rides your lady's brain and other vital organs at about the time in which it's most advantageous for her to get pregnant. Half time. (Though for the little boys who didn't bring their permission slip to that special class, pregnancy is possible for many days before ovulation, it just gets more so as ovulation approaches. Make a note of it.)

But relax. We have birth control. So, it is the wise man who does not ignore the *half time show*. If you like show girls, buy her a thong and feathers. And it is this time when she'll be most likely to come running at you wearing them. (And slam and head-butt you if you don't pay her some attention.)

3rd Quarter, a steady pace resumes.

4th Quarter, prepare yourself…

Last half of the 4th quarter…hunker down.

PMS has entered the game like a last minute addition by the coach of the meanest, orneriest, (yet surprisingly tidy) player on the team, to carry you through the last moment on the clock. Got it?

Let's review the play-by-plays.

First, picture your high school coach throwing his finger in the face after practice, quizzing you about what you've learned. Answer as quickly as possible. Imagine you won't have to shower with that big guy named "Ricky" if you get the right answers, cause coach will let you go change immediately.

(Hold the answers upside down to see if you're right.)

Kick off!?   *Day 1—menstruation starts*
How many plays/days to a 4th down?—*About four—Flo leaves the field*
Ovulation!? *Day 14 – half time hornies*
Last minute of play?! Last day – end of game—major PMS !
                                        You're really doing this?

See. You *can* get these minor complexities. Now, we can proceed with the rest of the book. You'll now have some idea of what I'm talking about when I say, "Play Ball!" And no, there are no special chapters devoted to half time exclusively. So don't bother thumbing back to the contents to see if you can just skip the rest. It's all important.

You might have noticed this is a particularly short chapter. Football deserves no more discussion here.

Chapter 3

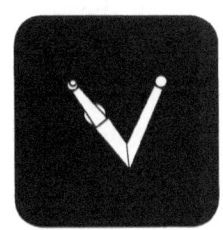

Cramps

It is the aim of this chapter to enlighten you about the delicate complexities of monthly pain. We want you to be educated, aware and above all, able to spot a convenience store likely to carry Motrin from at least 300 yards.

This is for your own good. Because if you can't, you'll be required to execute U-turns at 67 mph. And the rear tire has already been slashed in response to your witty repartee' about "aspirin being able to do the trick."

The history of cramps.

It is believed that the first cramp was indeed felt by Eve, as punishment for the apple scenario. Long lost scrolls recently discovered in Syria have revealed that Noah only saved female species, which exhibited cramps. The wise Noah did this knowing that the animals which would shoulder the burden for re-inhabiting the entire planet would have to have a guaranteed sex break for at least a few days at a time.

So, as you can see, cramps are a completely natural, albeit unpleasant phenomenon, which have served a useful purpose in our evolutionary development over the centuries. We as an advanced culture, however, are still completely baffled as to what that purpose could possibly be.

Therefore, we have come to the scientific conclusion that cramps are simply the work of Satan. Apparently, during creation, he created a series of evil accomplishments over a period of three days instead of six.

One the first day, he created mood swings, and it was bad.

On the second day, he created cramps, and it was worse.

On the third day, he created the first British cooking school. And birthed the oxymoron.

His work was done.

Modern Medicinal Assistance.

We've come a long way in the medical treatment of cramps. Today's environment of preventative medicine, cleaner living, better diet, and holistic approaches to health have made it abundantly clear that the treatment of cramps can be aided through the regular and systematic use of serious drugs. Ibuprofen has been the aid of choice among millions of women, for several years now. There are various brands available at your local drug store. Just ask the bagger at the checkout, which are best. He'll know as well as I.

Some of their over-the-counter brand names include:

Motrin—The "original" Ibuprofen.

Advil—A blue label, for the woman who's a "Winter" or "summer" color wheel

Nuprin—A bright, yellow label, easy to spot from way over at the tampon aisle.

Sunshine Label, also called, "brown coated tablets", or "Plain Wrap" (Brought to you by the same entity that offers plain wrap green beans, plain wrap cereal and plain wrap turkey sausage. Have no fear.)

Utilize these medications only after consulting a physician, *and* thoroughly studying the small, 14-page leaflet of warnings folded the size of a small spit wad and crammed in the bottom of the box. These medications are ingenious medical breakthroughs in so far as the average woman will spend a good 2 days intently focused on attempting to remove the little glued foil over the top of the bottle, *and* on removing the wads of cotton fiber from it's interior. We'll invariably then go in search of a tweezers for assistance, which we can't find in this mess of a bathroom, which will, in turn, beget a cleaning rampage of said bathroom, until three days later in which the tweezers have been found, and the cramps are gone.

Just in case you do actually break through the seals and cotton… most of the bottles will have handy instructions for use, as well as a lengthy list of warnings to frighten you from ever actually taking the medication and therefore, needing the instructions. We believe these lengthy warnings are a clever attempt on the part of the pharmaceutical companies to merely make the cramps seem "not so bad after all," in comparison to what sound like nasty, dreaded complications of actually taking the pills, or of mixing them with other dangerous compounds, such as Los Angeles area tap water.

Most directions state the following:

Directions; Adults Take 1 tablet every 4 to 6 hours while symptoms persist. If pain or fever does not respond to 1 tablet, 2 tablets may be used but do not exceed 6 tablets in 24 hours, unless directed by a doctor. But all 6 tablets in the same one of the 24 hours is a big no-no. The smallest effective dose should be used. By smallest effective dose, we mean to simply look at the bottle, and see if symptoms persist. If so, and you insist on actually *taking* this medication, take with food or milk if occasional and mild heartburn, upset stomach, or stomach pain occurs with use. This is a perfectly normal reaction as a nervous stomach is very common when taking medications after having actually read the warning leaflet. Consult a doctor if these symptoms are more than mild or if they persist. By "persist" we mean if they last longer than 2 or more minutes. Children: Do not give this product to children under 12 except under the advice and supervision of a doctor…who will charge you the traditional $347.97 "label-reading fee" —who will then prescribe this medication to you in handwriting so illegible, you will not know it's supposed to be this medication. And you may likely wind up taking a suppository for tapeworms and toenail malaria.

Active Ingredient: Each tablet contains Ibuprofen USP 200 mg, SPF 15. And eye of newt. See consumer information leaflet for complete directions and warnings. (That means there's more.)

Today's open acceptance of the need for pain treatments to aid women suffering from menstrual cramps is in sharp contrast to the medical opinion prevalent in our mother's generation. In previous decades, women who complained of abdominal cramping were told the pain was in their head...this, while these women lay curled in a fetal position on the waiting room floor busily growing fangs.

The favored response among many women of the time was to staple the lips of the doctor shut, blacken both eyes, then tell the doctor the pain in his head was really in his nuts.

Thankfully, it was soon the 60's, and so many doctors had their lips stapled in response to their theories, however, that serious studies of the cramping phenomenon were soon undertaken.

These studies proved, conclusively, once-and-for-all, that cramping hurt. And now that we've made this medical breakthrough it's time for pharmaceuticals to take over. (See the previous over-the-counter medicine list.)

Once the pain relieving medications have been swallowed, here is a list of some items to remove from her sight, to aid in the pain relieving process:

Pantyhose.

Belts.

Birthing videos.

Now that you're thoroughly baffled, we'll move on to an even more baffling exploration of the specific qualities of cramps. Perhaps you have some questions.

What do cramps feel like?

Scientists in Rochester, Nevada have been attempting to uncover exactly what it is that causes menstrual cramps. After exhaustive study, they have recently concluded, "menstruation". Fortunately, they have also utilized their study, made up of thousands of interviews with suffering women, to scientifically describe the sensation of cramping phenomenon as feeling like:

A sumo wrestler bear-hugging your uterus.

These scientists have evidently been walking into moving doors, because anyone knows a sumo wrestler doesn't "bear" hug. But, our tax dollars must go *somewhere*. Nevertheless, we must be understanding, because the specific pain of cramps is indeed difficult to describe. I will therefore, give you a completely unbiased, inaccurate and unscientific improvement upon their description, here:

Cramps are an unusually acute yet generalized pain, involving sort of the abdomen, but deeper than that, not a stinging pain, but more like the soreness of a cut after surgery—but worse, and not a sharp pain, more like a dull ache—but worse, and not a lot of moving small pains, a constant, relentless one. Sort of. There.

It's like a sumo wrestler hugging your uterus.

The most recent studies by these top scientists in our nation's capital have also concluded: Women do not like pain.

For example, it has been my experience that I would prefer standing naked next to Elle on the Tonight Show than experience yet another bout of menstrual cramps. To put it in more male-centric terms, *you'd* probably prefer standing naked next to Elle on the Tonight Show (realizing she'd probably be laughing at you, look at that belly resting under this book), than experience menstrual cramps. It's that bad.

What can you do?

Knowing that men often need to be "Mr. Fix-It", I assume you're probably wondering what you can do to help, so rest assured. You can be of assistance. You've just got to get creative.

For example, there is a small town in Massachusetts in which the citizenry has taken it upon itself to enlist and organize a community-cramping brigade. At the sound of an alarm in town square, this entirely volunteer organization, springs into action, forming a human chain, much like a bucket brigade, passing Ibuprofen to the household in emergency need, putting out their fire, if you will.

The local divorce rate has since plummeted.

You too, can help. Just think "outside the box", if you'll pardon the expression.

When do cramps start?

Only when you're out of Advil.

Actually, for most women, cramps normally occur at the beginning of the cycle, (see chapter 2, "Kick off"), not just before. However for some lucky ladies, it precedes the event.

When do they stop?

At around age 46-52. But by then, you'll be running up extremely high air conditioner bills, and you'll have a whole new set of problems.

There are a few other things you need to know. Women, on the whole, feel about as feminine during this time, as your nearest Teamster. And you, being the thinking man, will no doubt use this time to approach us for sex.

Once.

If you're a slow study, perhaps twice. And if you're buying this book because you really don't get it, I'm afraid you can't be helped.

Women can do very little in the way of manual labor during this sensitive time. We can however, shoe shop via the Spiegel catalogue, if the cordless phone is within reach of the hand not actively clutching the abdomen. So, keep said catalog handy, for our sakes.

Also, a good backrub can do wonders. Not for the cramps, but for the relationship. Do it at half time, and all time-outs. We suffer. So should you.

Lastly, on the days your lady is cramping remember: this is an especially good time to start a new, independent hobby, such as woodworking. You could practice, for instance, by boarding up the bedroom door. With her inside.

Chapter 4

Cleaning

Why the cleaning fixations during this period? Once again, we must look at history and evolution.

Let's start with psychologists. Many of these professionals, who's names all start with Dr. and who have extremely intimidating credentials from many years at expensive universities, have concluded that the phenomenon of excessive cleaning during this time of the month, is actually the manifestation of a woman's "nesting" behavior. "Cleaning" is actually "nesting". We must remember that these learned doctors who spent so many years in school spent many years with their knees crammed underneath desks that are too small for any human larger than say, a Barbie doll, and as a result, had much of the circulation cut off between their lower and upper extremities resulting in their apparent lack of good judgement. Why else would they spend so much time in school. Their conclusion about "nesting", however, is sound.

Cleaning as nesting.

Nesting is of course a behavior with deep roots in our psychological and animalistic evolution. In fact, it began as far back as cave man days, as you might imagine.

Man: Where are all my mastodon parts?
Woman? Those old things? I threw them out.
Man: But I was saving those!
Woman: Oh, go clean the garage. I'm nesting.
Man: We don't have a nest. Or a garage.
Woman: Then build one.

And so it began. (Man's quest for tools.) And woman's constant requirements that the garage be tidy.

So as you can see, without a cyclical "nesting" period, our homes today would be filled with mastodon parts, the result of you guys hanging onto junk from your father's father's father's father. And his mastodon.

In later, more civilized periods, women still threw away things, but by this time, men had finally developed the "garage" which has, evolutionarily speaking, become the last "junk safe zone" a boundary which most women will not cross, even while hormonally challenged. After all, if we could actually clean the garage, we would have to admit to being able to find it.

Today, we women throw away the unimportant things, such as your college diploma and stock certificates, leaving room for the really important stuff, such as our cosmetics, and the multitude of sample lipsticks we get "free" with the purchase of a make-up bag for just $2,411. 03 at Macy's.

Practical Product Tips

At one time or another, you have no doubt been confronted by your wife wielding a can of some toxic cleaning substance. Know now that this need to use a highly toxic product such as "Pine-Off" or "Flesh-Away with Scrubbing Enzymes" is genetically embedded in our make-up. How else would we get the *Nature's Face, Summer Bronze,* all-natural, hypoallergenic, pure n' gentle, "lip blush" stain off the bathroom sink?

A woman has a special relationship with the cleaning products of her choice, a relationship not to be messed with when her nesting instinct reaches PMS fever pitch. Of this you must be aware.

One of your major responsibilities during the nesting phase will be to ensure there are plenty of cleaning supplies handy, lest your lady decide to use your toothbrush to excavate the roach poison from behind the pantry.

Therefore, you should be up to snuff on a few of the basics:

Supplies You'll Need:

1. Bleach
Commonly known as: the stuff in the big white bottle too heavy to actually load from the shopping cart to the car, so it sits on the shelf 'til the next shopping trip.

Recognizable by: the smell, which, under prolonged exposure, will completely excavate the interior of your nasal cavity, without rubbing or scrubbing.

Used most often to: prop up the garage door (see large bottle concept above)

Advertised as able to: "make colors brighter." The theory is, that by whitening the surface of whatever it is applied to, the reds, though now closer to white, will seem "more red". Proctor and Gamble clearly have a finely honed sense of corporate reverse psychology. That, or the original ad guy couldn't type, and "lighter" became "brighter."

2. Steel Wool
Commonly known as: grey scouring pads so good for cleaning that once done cleaning with them, they will leave a rusty stain.

Recognizable by: the low, low price tag. No other cleaning product is quite so affordable, except for say, bleach…which we already know you can't carry home.

Used most often to: prop up the uneven corner of the old garage refrigerator

Advertised as able to: scour the most stubborn goo from anything.

So good at removing "tough stains" it actually removes a good portion of the item itself, which was stained in the first place. A four-quart stockpot can be easily reduced to a decorative teaspoon in as little as one application.

3. Baking Soda

Commonly known as: the white stuff in the orange box, sitting open in the back of the fridge.

Recognizable by: the fact you never use it.

Used most often to: occupy space in the fridge.

Advertised as able to: deodorize the fridge, if left sitting open in the back. The lazy person's way to never clean the fridge. Recommended ad slogan: "If things are green and fuzzy, use some white and fluffy". (Don't try this at home. I am a professional ad person.) Most consumers however, are completely unaware of its many other uses, which were edited from the commercials, due to the fact these commercials could only be 30 seconds long. However, a good box of baking soda can also be used to occupy space in your pantry, your bathroom cabinet, your closets, and if truly needed, your garage.

4. Sponges

Stock up on both the cleansing *and* contraceptive types. Nothing is quite as attractive to your lady at this crucial time as an instant birth control method which includes foaming bubbles she can actually, "see working."

5. Rubber Gloves

Commonly known as: well, duh.

Recognizable by: 5 fingers. (On our planet)

Used most often to: protect a woman's hands while carrying away a box containing and entire roll of paper towels used to squish the spider contained within them.

Advertised as able to: soften your hands while you do dishes.

Get these products gentlemen. You will need them.

A word about labels…

When utilizing any of these cleaning products, please please please read the labels! For God's sake, these are not children's toys! You cannot use them Willy-Nilly. However, if your name is not Willy or Nilly, you can.

Labels are there for your own good…to serve as a constant reminder that you don't read them. If you were to read them, however, you would discover that the product in your hand could do *anything*, if only it were safe to do so. Use caution. Labels typically read something like this:

WARNING: This product, though advertised as being able to remove your bathroom walls without scrubbing, would, if used, actually remove all skin except that on the soles of your feet. In fact, it's amazing this bottle is intact.

Remember, these are dangerous products we're putting in the hands of a hormonally-challenged woman, so just stand back, lest she allow *you* to use some of them, which could be worse.

Pay Special Attention…

When the cleaning/nesting phase hits, know you will have additional responsibilities. It will also be your duty to steer your partner towards cleaning tasks which will be less detrimental to your marriage.

This handy chart should help to illustrate the gravity of the situation, should you not actively participate and keep her focused.

1. Remember, with just a Saturday afternoon and an extra hour, she can choose to clean:
A) The tub   B) your tool box

2. Or, faced with a Monday evening and Melrose Place in re-runs, she can organize:
A) under the kitchen sink B) Your check register

3. In as little as ten minutes, she can scour
A) The Toast R' Oven   B) Your engine block

4. With virtually no notice, she can be tempted to try "Lytex Fungal Foam" on:
A) The bathroom tile   B) Your guitar amp

At this point you may be wondering if your mate is really that affected.

For further clarification, take this handy quiz to help estimate the severity of her condition.

1. When the PMS "nesting" phase reaches a fever pitch, your lady cleans:
A) the tub…while you're bathing
B) her teeth

C) the dishwasher. Not as in, "cleaning out the dishes", but rather cleaning out the inside of the dishwasher, a particularly clean appliance.

2. When you're late for a dinner party, and she sees something messy:
A) She stops all forward motion for the door and straightens her hair
B) She re-sets her contact to be more accurately centered
C) She insists on getting in the car, if only to reach the "cleaning club" to pick up a vat of hydrogen peroxide and return immediately to that pig sty of an oven

3. When there's a coffee mug spot on the kitchen counter, she:
A) Wipes it up and finishes it off with hydrogen peroxide from question 2, above
B) Screams in terror
C) Hires a cleaning service Hazel would be proud of

4. When she sees a scene of desolation and destruction in a film you've rented, such as a scene from "Independence Day", she:
A) Shuts off the TV and proceeds to the fridge to find that box of baking soda and figure out something to do with it.
B) Covers her eyes and screams she can't look
C) Starts wiping the television screen *itself* with 409

5. There is a bird turd on your car window, and you're late to witness the birth of your sister's baby.
A) She pulls into the Hot N' Soapy $14.95 car wash behind 16 other Land Cruisers
B) She scrapes it off with a razor blade and Windex…on the shoulder of Interstate 10.
C) She insists you stop by the dealership to buy an entirely new vehicle

If you have more than three "C" answers, proceed immediately to chapter 10.

How to Help Her Clean. Or, the safe use of a full-strength fire hose.

The first thing you must accept is that it is impossible to really "clean" anything completely.

But she will try.

Do not try to get her to accept this, however, or we'll be revisiting Chapter 5.

For example, you may discover she feels the living room needs to be dusted. This, five minutes after "wiping it down" with a pre-dusting product. At this point, you can:

A) Tell her to clean something else and "you'll handle it" with a Q-tip in your hand and a dusting cloth which you frantically wipe with every time she enters the room so as to convince her you are indeed cleaning, or...

B) Remember that if she does clean something else, it could be your wrench and socket set, so you quietly let her resume the "dusting" thing, or...

C) Pick up the remote and click through multiple channels, exclaiming, "It's important to periodically clean the circuits inside the television mechanism, by rapid-firing through a variety of channels for a period of time, kind of like warming up the engine on the car to get the oil distributed."

But again, it is impossible to really clean anything. There are always some microbe-sized stephlocoqulembacilli left behind, which are invisible to the naked eye, but which, if we *could* see them, would look like giant, hairy, gray lobsters with teeth, which inhabit the cracks between the floorboard and the carpeting in the back corner of the den behind the file cabinet... or your eyelid. *This* is what she's after.

You see, the problem is, she's seen that National Geographic photo in which this creature is photographically blown up 13,462 times its real size, and it's beyond disgusting. The solution? Throw away your National Geographics and tell her that this creature is the *good* microbe, and only thing on earth which can actually destroy the *bad* microbe which looks like a giant, hairy, gray cockroach with teeth and an extra set of arms on its back, and it, if not destroyed by the *good* microbe, will actually occupy crevices deep within her ear.

She'll buy a lot of Q-Tips, start leaving treats behind the file cabinet, and the next thing you know, PMS is over. If this doesn't work, you *will* indeed need to learn how to use a full-strength fire hose. Keep this book for handy reference.

Step one:
Ask a fireman for his hose.
Step two:
Post bail.
Step three:
Buy your own fire hose at a do-it-yourself center
Step four:
Hose down the interior of your home taking care not to get the carpet wet. This will only attract more dirt, as your lady will explain.
Repeat, deleting steps one and two.

Which brings us to…

"Dusting" versus "picking up" versus "cleaning"

At this point, it's important you realize that by these three terms, we mean three entirely different things. *Dusting* is a wipe down of what may already appear (to an amateur) to be a perfectly tidy room. By Amateur, we mean you. "Tidy" is actually a big lie. During PMS, we know that the room is actually a cesspool of contaminants, which obviously include the microscopic, hairy, gray cockroach-with-teeth mentioned previously. What you may not realize is that these contaminants namely, dust, must be wiped down hourly.

"Picking Up" is of course, another task entirely. Picking Up is something you might do before you mother comes over. That is, remove all the beer cans, laundry, pizza boxes, and scraps of paper such as unpaid utility and mortgage bills, and cram them into the space behind the TV. This phenomenon is one most commonly exhibited at every other time *besides* PMS. It's not likely to rear its childish head when PMS is in full swing. Nay. During PMS, we might not "Pick Up" at all. It's more important to scour and cleanse behind the piles of debris than it is to remove them. That my friend, is "cleaning."

What I've cleaned

It has been my experience that without PMS, (or at least my cleaning lady), I would have to get a medical license so as to keep my own supply of Penicillin handy should friends stop in for a visit. And, I'd probably have to use a lawn mower to cut a pathway to my door—straight through all the Ed McMahon offers that can't be thrown away, lest he come to said door.

Fortunately though, PMS keeps this all in check.

Once, while late for a dinner date, I noticed, for the first time ever, the spaces between the wooden slots on my coffee table. Do you know this can be utterly filthy? And nothing fits in there! You spray 409, and all it does it liquefy the dirt and send it dribbling around. You can't really get anything in there to wipe it away. It's maddening!

I eventually simplified the job, by throwing the entire table away. This was of course, the next morning. But when I suggested breakfast in lieu of dinner, my date was not amused. He did invite me to clean his place, however.

My other favorite "cleanse" took place on a camping trip. That lovely spring holiday in Yosemite will be one I always remember…especially for the light-hearted reaction I had to the third day of *no shower*. I believe such a reaction is called, "pitching a fit". You see, the need to clean everything excessively during PMS, can extend to our very person, as it did on this trip. Fortunately I was camping with female friends, who naturally understood, as we soon became cyclically in-synch, (the subject of another chapter), and were repelling bears in unison.

It began rather unexpectedly. I had no idea that upon waking that third day to the chirp of birds and the refreshing smell of crisp mountain air, that I would suddenly leap from my sleeping bag, growl at my friend next to me, grab a wet-nap, towel and dish soap and run screaming into the camp latrine. A half-hour later, my friends entered to witness the sponge bath that had ensued, and the friendly Ranger explaining that the Doh-Boy pool would have to go because it blocked the entrance. My sobs were audible.

It all comes full circle

No doubt, at one time or another, you've found your lady in a frantic cleaning fit. You console. You try to help. You get out of the way. You move to Montana. Then you realize, she'll only find you there because you packed a dirty suitcase, which she must track down and clean. So, you buy a new one and move to Hawaii, which has many more people inappropriately, dressed, and you'll blend in better. But she knows that by now your underwear is dirty, so she still finds you. You move home. And try to think of another plan next week. It's a cycle for all of us.

You see, this entire cleaning, or "nesting" phenomenon, is temporary, for most women. So fear not. Our contents of our make-up bags will soon be strewn across the bathroom. Our pantyhose will be hanging on the shower. And your dishes can remain stacked on the coffee table where they belong. Just learn to be patient. This should happen at about menopause.

Chapter 5

Mood Swings.
OR, *The many facets of a finely cut diamond*

It has been my experience, and perhaps yours, that PMS mood swings are the most insidious of the PMS symptoms.

A single word over dinner can mean the difference between a pleasant discourse and a nasty, downward-spiraling one. (Words such as "please", "napkin" and "bacteria" can be especially problematic. The reasons are obvious. Therefore, do not say anything.)

This will, of course, instigate a weeping bout over your insensitivity and your "emotional unavailability." This will pass as soon as dessert is served, and will be better than the alternative weeping over that obnoxious, "Please pass the salt"... request you may have otherwise carelessly carelessly uttered.

You see, translated, "Please" is a word you've *clearly* chosen to remind her that she's currently very sensitive. It is as if to say, "You're out of control—won't you, just for this instant *please* consider being human?" "Pass" is of course, your thinly veiled attempt to accuse her of being violent, (as if she were to "throw" it if you weren't specific) when it's perfectly obvious the salt is already within your reach. "The" is, of course in reference to your typical insistence that not just *any* salt will do, and of course, you use that special inflection in your voice as you say, "salt" to imply that we're retaining so much water this month, we remind you of The Big Fig Newton.

You see, the emotions of PMS are highly tuned. We are not, "out of control" as it may appear. We are actually at our most highly emotionally evolved. We can read the "truth" of every situation keenly. It's as if our sensor rays have reached super-human potential. We know what you are thinking. And we know what you really mean.

This power is dangerous, however, so we are limited to exercising it for only a few days out of the month, or, our species would not survive. That is why you must learn to camouflage your meanings, much like you would if you were to protect yourself from Superman's x-ray vision.

PMS Mood Swing, or the regular kind?

The best way to recognize a PMS mood swing is to note what the stimulus was for the mood's changing. If for example, your lady suddenly bursts into tears in response to an old Partridge Family episode, you could be facing PMS. Unless of course, it's the one where Shirley sings to the whales. That would make even Mr. Kincade cry. How could they spend money and time on such a stupid episode?

The hormonal shifts required to enable a woman to shed vital internal portions of her body, are designed to make her painfully aware that she is shedding vital internal portions of her body. Under the throws of tumultuously fluctuating hormones, a woman is likely to respond to stimuli tumultuously. Translated, this means Mood Swings are not our fault.

The duotwadinum and subcutaneous paleolithic layer of our mortification response must interact with the cumulonimbus lining, producing massive hormonal changes, not unlike those of the Incredible Hulk.

I'm sure you've witnessed news reports proving that too much rain in too short a time can flood the entire state of Oklahoma. We are talking about a downpour of hormones, which could easily cause your lady to clean the entire state of Oklahoma.

There are four basic emotions in the PMS repertoire. They may come in any order, or be paired with various subtleties. However, these "basic four" predominate:

Anger.

Glee.

Sadness.

Ennui².

Anger—most easily recognized by a propensity to redden in the face while "talkin sass." This sassing can even be in response to a television character, such as Amanda on Melrose Place reruns. The bitch.

Glee—recognizable by incessant laughter. When she finds the latest episode of, "Saved by the Bell" rather funny, you're in deep.

Sadness—often manifested by significant weeping, even at acts of kindness... like for instance, the mailman actually putting the flag up on your mailbox.

Ennui—a pervasive indifference, disinterest, and sense of hopelessness. Not unlike that which she may express at other times of the month when you insist on going tool shopping. (From the French term "ui"(wee), meaning bored, like you are.)

Mood swings have been a PMS tradition ever since Eve first experienced a hormonal craving and told Adam, "Get me something forbidden," then burst out again with, "It's not my fault! Fruit has no fat and I already look hippy!" Whereas *that* change in emotion was completely understandable, often, Mood Swings sneak up on your lady more subtly.

To put it another way, mood swinging is the phenomenon in which one emotion, (an emotion which the female host seems perfectly comfortable or natural manifesting), can suddenly and without warning shift dramatically to yet another, often unexplainable emotion.

It has been my experience that Mood Swings feel like the schoolyard game of "whiplash". In this game children link arms in a long line, then run around, changing direction so violently that Stinky Steve in the back gets whipped to and fro until his arms dislocate and he barfs on the baseball diamond, earning a whole new nickname. It's like crack-the-whip.

This is of course, the perfect Mood Swings analogy, not because of the whipping changes in direction, but because when I have mood swings I'm usually clenching my teeth at people and giving myself a headache, much like the headaches I used to get from laughing at the expense of other children in the schoolyard.

So, to understand Mood Swings, I will attempt to illustrate the most common/possible "swing" configurations for you here:

Anger-to-glee
This mood swing is characterized by its apparent mimicry of schizophrenia.

Whereas the initial anger may be situationally understood, possible initiators of the Glee shift may include Larry, Moe and Curly. This is the one and only time in which their violent-prone humor may work its special magic on a hithertofore uninterested female.

Other possible initiators of this mood swing might include, running out of gas...then discovering that you're in front of Boris' House of Biggie Burgers.

Or, if you're really desperate to *force* that glee shift from your Angry lady, invite

Uncle Harry over to tell another one of his Rabbi, Priest, Nun jokes after a bad Thanksgiving dinner, and she will laugh hysterically. This is a normal situation. Uncle Harry is hilarious. Not because of his jokes, because you notice once again that he always wears polyester pants with Nikes, so as to look "casual" and "ready for fun". She has to laugh.

Glee-to-sadness

Often the next immediate shift after Anger-Glee. This shift can arise most unexpectedly, such as when the Moe, Larry, Curly movie ends. And it becomes obvious that nothing's really funny. Nothing's ever been funny. And nothing ever will be again. Those brothers really love each other. The eye poking is just a ruse. And didn't she wish she were as close to her girlfriends these days as those three, good-natured, yuk-em-ups obviously are. Cheryl never calls. She's too busy with her new job. And Carlene has always been jealous..perhaps *she* needs a big poke in the eye…

…which brings us to:

Sadness-to-Anger

It doesn't take long for the sad woman to become angry. Sadness is passive…lonely…introspective…and self-reprimanding. In short order, the PMS'd woman will instead find someone to blame. Even if it is you. After all, there usually *is* someone to blame.

You may see this one coming, however, if you pay close attention to her "tps" or tears per minute quotient. (Mentioned in chapter One). It is when this quotient is at its peak that the change will occur. Absolutist words such as "never", "always" and "no one", are indicators of the *big switch* as well. You want to know, because phrases such as, "You never hold me," "I'll always be fat," and "It's never going to be Tuesday…" can serve you in this crisis. Immediately remove any angering objects, such as yourself, from the room.

Sadness-to-Ennui'

In more rare instances, sadness can dissipate into indifference. Indifference about work. Ennui' about relationships. Even an unwillingness to take action, such as the action of actually pulling forward at a green light. In her mind, there's time...and, it doesn't matter anyway.

Ennui-to-Anger
One of the more subversive mood swings. Ennui' can lull you into a false sense of security. Much like a good episode of Saturday Night Live. You think you're okay. PMS ain't so bad. She's even letting you woodwork without fussing about the mess everywhere. Then it hits. The Anger switch is usually preceded by her discovery of the lint in your pockets. Lint which clearly is the result of your placing tissues in there. When she's clearly told you not to.

So now, you should be discovering clear, very sensible, and obviously instigated transitions. My solution? Hide your pants.

Glee-to-Ennui'
Probably the most harmless of the typical mood swings, unless of course, you're on a game show. This swing can be very detrimental. Imagine if you will, spinning the big wheel, having 3 seconds left on the clock to name any one of the Brady Bunch, and your previously giddy wife decides $34,000 won't pay for college anyway.

It could happen.

You see, mood swings are all about a change in her perspective. Perspective is everything. If you were about to bleed for several days, wouldn't your perspective change? Things are amplified. Senses are finely honed. The little things take on new meaning, like, how the word *bear* can change in meaning from, "*carry*", to "*big grizzly.*"

THE PMS PERSPECTIVE—A CHART

SITUATION:	WHAT SHE SEES:
The neighbor's thumping again	She develops an intimate understanding of Edgar Allen Poe's Telltale Heart
You're late for dinner	You have obviously been sitting in a small room frittering away time discussing something trivial, say, for example, the situation in Bosnia, probably in the company of the same guy who cut her off in the bank parking lot earlier, and that blond you stumbled at the sight of during the Christmas party 5 years ago.
The tire looks flat	The Donut Shop is probably open
Afternoon Tea	H.Salt Fish 'N Chips has tea...
Her favorite book is missing	The necessity to rip the individual pages one by one out of every book she can find to teach the missing one a lesson
Star Wars, a classic fantasy/action/adventure	An emotionally wrenching, sob-inducing tour-de-force triumph of the spirit as evidenced by the deeply moving, touching, pre-dinner seen in which Luke makes friends with the adorable, R2-D2, a tragic mythic figure
You're out of toilet paper	The opportunity to substitute with a "Sears Finest" 100% cotton towel, then cram it, and likely every other towen in the cabinet, straight into the toilet and flush...a plot clearly spear-headed by that witch of a head cheerleader in high school, because there's <u>no</u> <u>toilet paper</u>, there's never any toilet paper, <u>ever</u>, an if there was, it would probably be that crumbly plain-wrap kind so why not just use typing paper anyway!
The VCR is blinking	A flashing neon high-beam of a MAC truck pulsating incessantly with an almost lifelike urgency, who's evil must be extinguished by any means necessary, not excluding the kitchen fire extinguisher. After all, it is alive.

There is one more deep, dark secret, I will share with you here. The shopping hormone is linked to the mood swings hormones. It cannot be helped. For centuries, women have carried this burden. It has evolved for our own good. Otherwise, the only relief we would enjoy once a month is food, which would leave us all 900 lbs. Thanks to the shopping hormone, we're just broke... but able to return things.

Once, while shopping for a new a new box of laundry detergent, I found myself instead purchasing an expensive pair of sassy pants, (defined as pants you could never wear outside of metropolitan Los Angeles or New York without being arrested). I did this all the while crying over how bad I looked in them. This also, cannot be explained. (The purchase, I mean. Not the crying. I was bloated.)

My older sister, not always known for consistency of mood, has gone to great lengths to prove this theory. Her closet is filled with expensive clothes, which prevent her budget from allowing for other extra-curricular activities, such as paying her mortgage. Shopping happens monthly, and food is not her strongest PMS craving. Hence, she is skinny and well dressed.

One final section:

If any of you men happen to be sitting smugly in a vat of self-satisfaction and social superiority, rather than marinating in sympathy, there is something you should know. It is a well-proven scientific fact that MEN suffer from the effects of wildly fluctuating hormones. They just experience it DAILY as opposed to monthly. So stick that in your pipe and smoke it.

In the same way that many women manifest the effects of fluctuating hormones, many men experience inexplicable tirades, traversing wildly from concern to anger.

I once had a boss, who, at the sound of a check being torn from the Accounts Payable ledger, would go into a door-slamming fit down the halls. A simple Hostess Twinkie, or visit from the big-busted intern would cheer him up. At least *we* try to keep the subjects of our rage rational, like the lint in your pants pockets.

The preceding notation was originally going to be the subject of an entirely separate chapter, entitled "So There" but, I refrained. I just felt a Swing from Angry to Ennui'.

Mood Swings Can Be Good.
They really can. Make the most of them. When you've been over-charged by the phone company, or your bank balance is incorrect, wait to check the calendar before you take action, and have your lady do it. She'll be amazingly efficient, leaving nothing but a small, well-trimmed piece of flesh behind, something like a skilled butcher would. Or, you may want to ask your wife to read that screenplay idea you've been keeping in the back drawer since college. She'll find it the most touching memoir of love and honor ever visualized for the screen. Your ego will soar. Never mind that it's an idea for "Bikini-clad Car Wash Girls in 3-D".

The Hornies.
Yup. Your eyes raced down here.

Well, the simple truth is, with hormones a-ragin', and moods a'swingin', some women (like me), can also get suddenly, and inexplica-bly horny at PMS time.

DANGER! DANGER! DANGER!
This is not always a good thing. Unless, of course, you don't mind being told how, why, and what to do. Every step of the way. Now. I mean, right NOW!!!!!

Hurry! Before I pinch your head off! You get the idea.

Water Retention.
One might wonder why mood swings and water retention have been associated in this chapter. Don't be silly. Anyone's moods are likely to be

sporadic when faced with an overnight weight increase of 22 1/2 pounds. This of course, has nothing to do with the potato chip/brownie sundae phenomenon. It's simply excess water.

Our breasts usually swell, often as much as 9 cup sizes. This of course causes the shopping gene to present itself, full force, wherein we rush to Victoria's Secret, spending countless hours trying on skimpy, lifting, pushing, lacy, racy undergarments in an attempt to comfortably fit this temporary blossom, leaving the store with a bag filled with only pot pouri. We couldn't possibly, actually *buy* any of those new things when our stomachs look so gross.

This is for the best, as one week later, many men across America are known to exclaim, "Honey, you shrunk your breasts!" after enjoying their tautness and fullness for days. At least it gives you something to look forward to.

Speaking of tautness and fullness, our water-retentive "blossom" is tender, and it requires a tender touch. Not that you're not the most skilled and sensitive lover we've only had, but, leave the vice grips in the garage. Honey. Or, Ms. Mood Swing may make a noticeable appearance.

Water retention, however, can be a highly upsetting condition, causing a woman to fixate on her swollen body. We're delighted with our breasts, and overwrought about our stomachs, which again plays right into the Ms. Mood Swing's hands. So proceed with caution.

Water retention is also a condition which can dramatically effect our sense of coordination and balance, because water retention is known to effect the brain and equilibrium. Fortunately, the shopping response can kick in, allowing us to easily replace whatever items we may have clumsily dropped, and find several new pairs of shoes with low heels, the better to balance on.

Now you understand.

WOMEN WHO HAVE NEVER HAD PMS :

WOMEN IN A CONSTANT STATE:

WOMEN WHO HAVE NEVER HAD PMS :	WOMEN IN A CONSTANT STATE:
Marcia Brady	Jan Brady
Divine	(Leona Helmsly remembers)
Eleanor Roosevelt	Alien
Joan of Ark	The French Lieutenant's Woman
Annette Funicello	Peg Bundy
Katie Curek	Nancy Reagan
Debbie Boone	The Pine Sol Lady
Mary Lou Retton	Tonya Harding
Miss Marriane	Hobo Kelly
Leah Thompson	Joan Crawford
Julia Childs	Betty Crocker

Chapter 6

Sex

Upside?
   1) Big boobs.
   2) Horny hormones.
   3) Impatience. ("I want it and I want it...NOW...DAMMIT!)
Downside?
   3) Mood swings likely to swing into action unexpectedly leaving you
      an ego-deflated heap of tired flesh. (see point #3, above)
   4) Possible Cramps. But the swollen teeth marks on your hand will
      keep you from even posing the question, if cramps do crop up.
      This is a dilemma which only you can resolve. Good luck.

Chapter 7

PMS in the Workplace

The author realizes that some of you men out there may actually work with your dearly beloved. Or, unless you're the Scout Leader at a back-woods militia camp, most of you work with at least some ladies. Which makes a knowledge of how PMS effects a woman's work performance as relevant as say, knowing how to spell your name, walk, or where to buy beer.

Let us take a moment to dispel some misconceptions about PMS and workplace functionality. You see, it is precisely at this time when a woman may be at her most productive.

In a scientific experiment conducted by scientists somewhere, it was discovered that pre-menstrual hamsters could spin the Habitrail wheel as much as 19 times faster than their non-pre-menstrual counterparts.

> *Scientist 1: Look at her go.*
> *Scientist 2: Yup. She's bookin.*
> *Scientist 3: Let's get another federal grant.*

It is also important to note here that women have the innate ability to do two or more things at a time. This trait dates back to caveman days, when women could often be seen nursing an infant, gathering roots, berries and tubers, and gossiping about Tondor's receding hairline, all while weaving small baskets with their teeth, (perfect for brightening up the cave entrance). What does this have to do with modern workday PMS? Plenty, my friend. It is while in the workplace that a woman harnesses this innate multi-tasking ability, and combines it with both the six-minute attention span (see chapter 8), and her

cyclical compulsion for order, in order to accomplish amazing feats. Tasks such as a complete corporate reorganization, the development of a computer chip that runs NASA (or the cosmetic counter's color-check computer), *and* the processing of zodiac horoscopes for all Boeing employees can be completed during this stage in record time.

For example, while working for a small ad agency in Santa Monica, California, it was during PMS that I completed campaign ideas for a 6 month period, re-decorated the offices, scoured the bathroom and appointed myself CEO. All before the 9:30 production meeting. I had arrived at 9:15.

At this point, the less savvy man may require some tips as to how to handle various pre-menstrual women in your work environment, with consideration given to their work relationship to you. The following scenarios should help.

FEMALE CO-WORKER AS SUBORDINATE

Here's the situation. You arrive at work. Suddenly and without warning, your Administrative Assistance tells you she's finished the coffee, copies and distributed the memos, pasted up the boards for your presentation, booked your flight and e-mailed your notes to the affiliates, all with your boss standing over your left shoulder.

Now you look really stupid because you couldn't do all this in a whole week, let alone one morning. The point is, you see the remnants of a "hefty burger" bag in the trashcan, a large diet soda, and a "party sized" bag of potato chips by her chair. You, the intelligent male, note the signs and react appropriately.

"Re-file everything. Write the annual report. Prepare my agenda. And create my next three presentations." Then, you immediately hand her the large bag of Frit-O-Lay somethings you have handy for this very occasion. NOTE: Do not mention anything else. DO NOT note the foodstuffs, stuffed under her chair. DO NOT ask how she's feeling. DO NOT say, "My, but you've been a busy bee" lest she believe you're noting that the rest of the time she's not nearly so productive. You will be sorry. Merely take action, and take advantage. Quietly. Next, require lots of quiet time with your door shut.

FEMALE CO-WORKER AS ASSOCIATE

Here's the situation. You arrive at work. Suddenly and without warning, your Associate tells you she's finished the coffee, copied and distributed the team memos, pasted up the boards for your joint presentation, booked her flight, and e-mailed your notes to the affiliates. All with your boss standing over your left shoulder. Now you look really stupid because you couldn't do all this in a whole week, let alone one morning. The point is, you see the remnants of a "hefty burger" bag in the trashcan, a large diet soda, and a "party sized" bag of potato chips by her chair. You, the intelligent male, note the signs and react appropriately.

"Excellent work. Why don't you put a few thoughts down about the annual report. Prepare our agenda. And start on the next three presentations." Then, you immediately hand her the large bag of Frit-O-Lay somethings you have handy for this very occasion. NOTE: Do not mention anything else. DO NOT note the foodstuffs, stuffed under her chair. DO NOT ask how she's feeling. DO NOT say, "My, but you've been a busy bee" lest she believe you're noting that the rest of the time she's not nearly so productive. You will be sorry. Merely take action, and take advantage. Quietly. Next, require lots of quiet time with your door shut.

WOMAN AS BOSS

Here's the situation. You're screwed. There's no possible way you can keep up with her productivity. Just plan to work late for four days each month to keep up appearances.

OTHER HANDY TIPS

It is precisely at PMS time that a woman may exhibit behaviors quite different from what you might normally expect in the workplace.

Whereas at any other time of the month, a woman might ask your opinion on a weighty issue, then, either:

A) Not listen to the answer (walking decisively toward another part of the room *while* you speak), OR

B) Not take the advice that she does indeed listen to.

At this time, however, she will not ask your opinion at all.

Consider it a reprieve.

The water-cooler scenario

Oftentimes, the water cooler offers a small oasis of social interaction in the work environment. Here, comrades can share a joke, catch up on the gossip or merely make some impromptu plans for the weekend. Know now that the PMS'd woman will be nowhere near here, because there's no sugar in the water, nor is there fat. Therefore, if any of your little social moments require her social interaction, just yell toward the office refrigerator on the other side of the room.

The Xerox machine scenario

You see the machine is malfunctioning. You quickly note that it may have something to do with the crow bar protruding from the gaping, steaming hole in its side. There is a nacho-cheese-smelling fingerprint on the blinking red button. Hm.

Should you:
A) Back away slowly
B) Call Xerox and inform them of this model's deficiencies
C) Scream loudly
D) Speak in obnoxiously loud tones to someone across the room about how *you* prefer regular to nacho cheese.

The only appropriate answer is A. How else will you be able to act truly non-challant when you inquire as to whether anyone has any junk food around when you want some of the chips?

This is an especially good time to practice copying materials for the office in long hand. Xerox has gotten very speedy with their repairs lately and will usually arrive within hours, which, is far too soon. Unless about 4 days elapse, the machine will be broken again immediately.

The order desk scenario

Customer service can be fraught with peril at this time. Not for the customer, for the PMS'd out woman. Do you know how many times we risk mascara runs when the computer printer sticks and makes crooked printouts? Which is obviously because we're unloved?

Sales woman: It won't print!
Orderer: Turn it on.
Sales woman: (weeping) I suppose you know the answer to everything…
Orderer: I know you gotta turn it on.
Sales woman: He hasn't even tried in three days.
Orderer: That's more info than I wanted…

The meeting scenario…

You may also find it necessary to participate in a particularly common office ritual, in which members of your company, some of whom appear to be complete strangers, gather in a small room with a large table. Soon thereafter, gossip is exchanged. Some members meander out for soft drinks. Eventually, though, they must proceed to the business at hand and discuss the previous episode of The Practice, and who is engaged to whom. (Not on The Practice, but at the office.) This is what has been referred to in some lofty business schools, as "the department meeting". Eventually, before adjourning, someone will discuss something of which you know nothing about, but which you will be more than happy to pontificate on, as is your duty in these gatherings. After going around the table and assessing everyone's personal opinions on the issue in the most irrelevant and minute detail, nothing is resolved.

Fortunately though, the guy from Accounting, who is most unaffected and uninformed about the subject, will stand up to discuss why it's not prudent to do this. Or anything. In fact, every course of action can be problematic from his point of view. Even thinking about one could be unwise. And he'll give you 137 reasons why. This is perfectly understandable. If you were an accountant, you would *live* for those moments in which you get to stand up and talk, if most of the time you were calculating the square root of the electricity bill.

So then, the issue is "shelved" until someone, somewhere comes back with more information, (usually defined as even more personal opinion on how the subject may effect them on the 3rd Tuesday of February, next year). How is this relevant to PMS? If any woman in the room is affected, the Accounting Guy gets a fork in his forehead. And you cheer. What did I say about being at our most productive? When the ambulance arrives, you get to sneak home early, during the chaos.

The vending machine scenario...

You enter the kitchen and discover the vending machine has nothing but Nature's Musk low-fat granola clusters. The Twinkies, Ding Dongs, Cheetos, Famous Amos, and Hershey bars are gone. Go home. Better to use your sick days on a day like this than one a day when you're actually sick and can't enjoy it.

The birthday cake scenario.

Oh, that time-honored tradition of pretending to surprise a co-worker with a birthday cake. This can be an especially convenient time to discover who's on their cycle. The woman who's already eating a Hershey's crackle when she steps up to the plate, could be a contender. Unless of course, she regularly does this. If the kitchen counter is lined with women, all holding their plates and forks, go home. There won't be a piece for you anyway. Or, if there is, it will be the size of a slice of bologna, hardly worth the rendition of "Happy Birthday" in Q flat, you had to endure to get here.

So you see, PMS can be productive situation in the workplace. Just make sure you don't sit next to that guy from Accounting in any department meetings.

Chapter 8

The 6-Minute Attention Span

One of the most interesting symptoms of PMS is the 6-minute attention span. I realize that this may be an extended attention span for some, (for example, those women who put on mascara on a freeway interchange), but for most of us however, it is a reduction. This is a scientific fact, which means again, that it is not our fault. It seems the very same chemicals which cause our bodies to shed vital interior contents, also cause us to shed hours from our sensory perception.

You see, our neurons are under stress. They've been told hormones are moving in, so they're nervous. They're in a constant state of readiness. To help you envision the scenario, imagine those times when your scary uncle is expected for a visit, and everyone's running around cleaning, hiding your piano, and putting the chips away, all the while jumping at every little motor that runs by outside. In much the same way, your lady's brain is rapid-firing frantic signals to her that something's coming, and she better *do something*…though she's not sure what it is.

Hence, you'll hear a lot of, "Huh?" "What?" and "Oh yeah," from her, much as we currently do from the extreme Senior Citizenry of our Supreme Court.

At this fragile time, your lady's attention can meander continuously between unrelated things. For example, she may sit at your outrageously expensive home computer (which you do not use except to play *Death Warriors in Leather Bras*), and express a desire to begin her authoring of the Great American Novel, so as to put the pricey Nintendo to good use. Suddenly, she seems utterly fascinated with her navel lint, and soon thereafter, begins to scour the kitchen sink.

By the end of the evening, she's typing with one rubber glove on, while a pile of lint sits next to the "escape" key, but the words she's processing on the screen read, "where are the Doritos?" This is perfectly normal. Anyone who's ever tried to write the Great American Novel gets distracted by their navel.

If your lady does the cooking in your relationship, this can be an exceptionally good time to enjoy entirely different dining experiences such as:

Stouffer's Lean Cuisine (microwave time: 5 1/2 minutes)
Jello "instant" pudding
The 3-minute egg (fried)
Cheese
Instant Oatmeal
The Taco-Man drive-through. (served in 2 minutes or it's free!)

Nature is kind. Our cravings for this crap coincide with their brief preparation requirements. There's so much symbiosis, it's really amazing.

How It Works

It may help you to understand the limited attention factor, by illustrating for you how the actual attention process works in her mind.

For example, perhaps you've gone shopping for a few essentials at the local "Bulk o'Rama" store. First, make sure you take the sport utility vehicle. Nothing they sell will fit in anything else. Next, bring a book for reading in the check out line. Then, you actually make a list of the items you need.

1. the 52 cup coffee pot
2. Fruit Loops in the economy 9 pack
3. the 48 slice toast r' oven
4. tires

Once you arrive, you suggest heading for the coffeepots first. And the scenario goes something like this:

Your Beloved: Sure. Coffee pots.
(She stops and picks up a Dr. Seuss pop-up book.)
You: Honey, the coffeepots?
Your Beloved: We should put one on our list next time.
You: We did.
Your Beloved: Yup.
You: They're on aisle 12
Your Beloved: Do these pants make me look hippie?

What really happened:

The moment she entered the store, your mate's mind fixated on the yellow vest of the person checking your Bulk 'o Rama membership cards. This would of course, cause her to remember the old brown vest in the bag of clothing she needs to take to the Good Will, which, when she does, will invariably mean she has to walk by the cranky woman at the back gate who's pregnant, and who reminds her that not every child gets a good parent, but fortunately, her friend Mimi's baby will have exceptional parents in as much as both Mimi and her husband adore children, and often remind her of her cousin Elena, who also loves children and who swears by reading to them. Then, she sees the Dr. Suess display, which has nothing to do with the aforementioned thoughts.

However, she is in a simplistic state of mind so the cartoon graphics appeal to her and she grabs a book.

When you remind her of the coffee pots, she is on page 12...the page that reads,

"His hat was soft and green as lime.
He was a not guilty of a crime,
I do not like this kind of rhyme,
…*we should put one on our list next time".*

She puts down the book and looks up to see a small child with bits of cheese & cracker appetizer samples smeared all over his shirt. Some deep instinctual urge compels her to find the Nacho Cheese crispies aisle where there will undoubtedly be a 40 pound bag waiting, the consumption of which will enlarge her swollen belly another 19 inches, but, perhaps strategic dressing will help. The right pants make a difference, don't they? Hence, the "do these pants make me look hippie?" query. It all makes perfect sense.

So you see, her limited and varying attention at this time of the month can be most distressing if you do not understand it. Or, if you actually believe this chapter.

I of course, do, and that's why I've used the 6-minute attention span excuse to put off any number of pressing tasks, and to excuse any achievement shortcomings. And, it's been very effective.

Ways I've put the 6-minute attention span to good use:

Taken up the guitar. Today, I can play "8 Days a Week" in three chords only. I do this monthly.

Taken up Sculpture. I own five packages of clay that are happily sitting in my closet. Perhaps next month, one of their plastic seals will be broken and I will actually sculpt something. Like an asymmetrical ball in one fist.

Taken up painting. I own a small set of watercolors. They will be wetted in about two months.

Taken up sewing. I have threaded my sewing machine.

Learned Bridge. I have bought a deck of cards.

Taken up Numerology. I have thought my name must have some number that means something attached to it.

Caught up on my reading. I have read the first 4 pages to 3 different highly regarded novels. Page-turners? Hah.

Organized photo albums. Those that I have purchased sit neatly organized by size, next to the mismatched piles of photos and negatives on the fireplace.

Cleaned dust from one of the three blades on my summer fan. It will take two more months to clean the other two. If I remember to do so.

Studied Spanish on audiocassette. "Hola. Mi llama es Kay. Muy Bue—muy bue—hey, donde estan last papas fritas?"

I'm being far too modest here. Actually, after 12 months of these six-minute bursts, I've actually learned the first *two* versus to "8 days a week". Not well. That would take another twelve months.

Can you recognize the six minute attention span?
How often does it rear its ugly head in your relationship? Have you attributed her behavior incorrectly to your merely being boring? To find out, take this handy quiz.

1. When she asks you a question, such as "how was your day?" does she walk away without listening to your answer?
   Don't worry. All women do that.

2. When you pop in a video of "Driving Miss Daisy" (which she selected at the store), does she ask, "What are we watching again?"
Attention deficit.

3. If you begin baking Cinnamon cookies, does she pull out the Paprika?
Not a problem. Paprika looks like Cinnamon. She's just a bad cook.

4. When she steps out of the shower and dries off, does she turn it back on and go in again?
Attention deficit.

5. When driving to a dinner party at a location she's been to 300 times, does she pass it up and miss it by a mile or ten?
Definitely attention deficit. Only you guys do that.

6. If she says she's tired, then asks if you want to go running…
Attention deficit.

7. Does she prance around in a thong, then ask if you'd like her in something else?
She's ovulating. (See "Scoring at half-time", Chapter 2)

8. After squishing a spider in a tissue, then reaching back to shut the screen door, does she look back at the tissue and blow her nose?
Call a psychiatrist immediately. Women do not squish bugs when you're around.

Recommended attention-deficit distractions: (OR, On the bright side…)

Do not be discouraged. Though there are many annoyances to this attention problem, it can be fortuitous too. There are several ways you can work this phenomenon to your advantage.

For example:

* You can actually slip a porno into your video selection at the counter, then, when you get home, tell her it was her idea.

* Ask, "What fart?"

* Say, "Thanks for cuddling with me hon," then go to sleep.

* Too bad we missed the Chamber Music."

* Remind her, "I *told* you it was poker night. I thought you were going to the movies?"

* Proclaim, "That was so nice of you to offer me a beer."

* Thank her for offering to go to the store for more beer. Do this, however, knowing she may return with sewing notions.

* Propose.

* If you don't agree with her career change, have her do all the prep work now.

This is *not* a good time to:

Garden
Build a house
Have sex. (Unless 6 minutes is your usual.)
Play Bridge

Play Monopoly

Watch Lawrence of Arabia

(all that sand combined with the increased salt intake will make her thirsty)

Hook up your modem.

(it is never a good time to do this yourself. Call your friend who takes his PC to ball games and have him do it.)

It *is* a good time to:

Play Shoots N' Ladders

Play Spin the Bottle. (But it gets really embarrassing when she can't remember who she wanted the bottle pointing at)

Wash a cup

Flip through the TV channels aimlessly

Try your favorite knock-knock joke

Questions and Answers

"How many things can hold her attention at one time?"

1, 342.

"How can I help her focus?"

Hot fudge.

"If she asks me a question, how can I tell she'll remember what I answer?"

Look deep into her eyes. Then write down your answer and stick it in her pocket. It may still not work, but when she does laundry and finds the note that says, "Antipasto and Pee Wee Herman" she'll go nuts. Enjoy your revenge.

"What types of things make it worse?"

Re-runs of I Love Lucy and Mary Hart's voice. We don't know why.

"If we must go out to a nicer restaurant, how can I get her to order?"

You can't. Order for yourself, then order for her secretly. By the time your main dish is served, she won't remember that she never ordered, and will merely set her menu aside and start porking.

"What types of sports can she do now?"

BBQ

"Is there anything else I should know?"

Try chapters 9-11.

"Is there a medication that will help?"

It's illegal now unless prescribed in certain states.

"My wife seems to exhibit this behavior 30 days a month."

You don't say how long you've been married. If it's after the 3rd week, that's normal.

"My girlfriend never remembers our phone number. What's up with that?"

Check if she knows the credit card number. If not, we're sorry. She's simply an idiot.

"Can I really pull off the "thanks for cuddling thing?"

Would I lie?

"Why must I know or care about the 6-minute attention span? It doesn't sound so bad?"

We realize that this personality trait merely reminds you of some of your best friends, like Louie, but, would you really want to live with Louie? Yes, gentlemen, *you* are usually the proud exploiters of limited attention, the rest of the time. But at this critical juncture, if you're both out-to-lunch, no one gets any. You will, *at this time,* have to cease the channel flipping, or nothing gets watched. Turn off the stove, or everything gets burned. Remember the directions, or you don't get there. And for God's sake, remember where you put your own keys for just a few days.

If you do not extend your attention span during this period when hers is weakened, especially if you are traveling, you're liable to end up with no car keys, no shaving kit, no airplane tickets, and no ultimate destination.

One Final Note

This is a time in which you simply must do your own laundry. Even if you do not have any. Otherwise, she will find *something* to wash. And, it will all be pink. It will also be either tumble-dried dirty, or washed three times in Super Clean n' Tidy Toilet Bowl Cleaner with scum-removing crystals. Or washed four times without soap of any kind. The possibilities are endless.

If, however, this is the way *you* usually do laundry, then fine. No love lost.

FAMOUS ACHIEVEMENTS PARTLY ATTRIBUTABLE TO THE PMS PHENOMENON

- The Storming of the Bastille (They thought "the cake" was there.)

- Inquisition Torture Devices (to simulate cramping for men)

- The Great Wall of China (nesting taken to an extreme)

- Stonehenge

- The first foot-long deli sandwich

• The Concept of "Biggie-Fries"

• The Alaskan Oil Cleanup

• Boston Tea Party (see item 4, chart 1)

• Midnight ride of Paul Revere (wife needed a late evening Haagen Daas with French Fries)

• 7 Dwarves Cottage, Spring Cleaning

• The invention of Simple Green

• The American Flag (Betsy Ross obsessed. Nuf said.)

Chapter 9

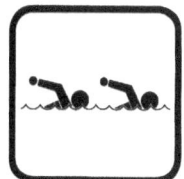

The Women-in-Synch Phenomenon

What happens when we live together? What happens when you live with several of us? Perhaps you have heard of the phenomenon of women whose cycles become synchronized when they spend a lot of time together, or live in the same household.

This is God's happy miracle. With more than one woman in your midst, you're spared a never-ending hormonal barrage. In other words, if you have 4 women in your company, you get to endure all of it simultaneously, at 4 times the volume.

My advice? Buy 4 books.

The Synching of the Cycles

Perhaps you've actually watched the History Channel and heard about how the American Indians would send all the women to the hills for a few days out of the month because they were all on the same cycle. This was when the first, "poker game with the guys" was invented.

A close friend of mine has also reported that many women on her soccer teams in various areas of Southern California have experienced the synching of their cycles. As of this writing, her league includes a buffet break and counseling for the players at half time during games occurring on third Tuesday of every month.

The knitting club that meets regularly at the VFW hall in Porcupine, New Mexico has been studied for several months now by the Center for Big Budget Hormonal Therapies Studies. It seems nine of these women's menstrual cycles are exactly synchronized. The tenth, Beatrice Lovenbraugh, is not, but this has been attributed to her crooked double half hitch and the resultant lack of acceptance by the other members of the group.

Conversations lately have gone something like this:

Mary: Ethel? You started yet?

Ethel: Due tomorrow.

Everyone: Me too! (In unison, which surprises all of them so much, they poke themselves with their knitting needles and all start swearing.) This has caused the Center for Big Budget Hormonal Therapies Studies to investigate eyewash, and has gotten them completely off the track… but there's always hope for the future.

Practical Tips.

First, clue-in. For instance, your wife *and* your daughter may both be experiencing cramps, bloating, food cravings, mood swings, short attention spans, and excessive tidiness at the same time, for perfectly natural reasons. You, being a male, may have for years found it perfectly natural not to notice. Well it's high time you did. When their hormonal activity is in synch, you the crafty male can schedule routine fishing trips, camping excursions, or at least a good nap in a more timely fashion. Just leave a tub full of cleaning products in full view by the door as you exit.

If you can't stand this double duty, and would rather take it in separate spurts, separate your wife and daughter. Two time zones should do the trick.

This is how the synch-up works…

First, a woman's ovaries smell other ovaries. The ovaries need to bond, much like we do in the bathroom. It's all connected.

First woman's ovaries: We're so different. No one is ever going to like us. Wait a minute? I smell something? It's very faint, but it smells just like me…Wow. Let's send out more pheromones to see if we can attract it over here. With any luck, we can all giggle together.

Other woman's ovaries: Hey….I smell something. Ooh. I think it's what we just finished. Damn. If that smell sticks around for a couple of days…we could make the hamsters run slower…maybe that other smell can catch up! With any luck, we can all go shopping together.

Finally, the glands all agree to set a new pace.

At this point, what begins to happen is what I like to call, The Snowball Effect. As soon as more than three women in the same vicinity synch, there is no stopping the surge of additional cycles, which gravitate toward one another. Multiple women's cycles inexplicably link up, and the energy grows, like The Blob.

That is why you should exercise extreme care and caution in various situations you may not have previously considered.

When interviewing for a job—

Note how many women are in the office. If the business is predominantly female, do not let the chipper, salad-eating demeanor of seemingly all of them distract you. Once a month, you could be facing French fry buffets and cake walks at closing, or, tirades about your lack of productivity. The elevator needs cleaning.

When shopping—

Consider this. It's time for you to purchase a gift for your lovely lady. Many of the mall stores from which she might enjoy a little something, are staffed *entirely by women*. For your own safety, browse casually near the window displays *before* entering. Note the general demeanor of the sales staff… Are they running around frantically, re-hanging every garment, and reminding you of ants in an ant farm rather than the charming Victoria's Secret employees that they are?

This would not be a good time to actually reveal your name and credit card number to any of them unless of course, you're very efficient about it. You should know exactly what you want and ask a minimum of questions like, "What size is this?" and, "How much do I owe you?" However, you might actually consider ignoring the "please no food or drink" sign, and bringing an offering from the food court, right up to the counter. If they dive on your Cinnebons like dingoes on a carcass, you could get a discount.

If, upon your initial investigation, they appear to be happily twisting their hair behind their ears, and reciting the same, "That's a really cute top" line to every customer who enters, enter freely, and have no fear.

Attending a Sorority Party—
That's disgusting. You're 38 years old. Don't even think about it.

Picking up your daughter from cheerleader practice.
The entire squad is hugging each other and crying. Either:
A) They just won the bouncy personality championships against 4 other schools
B) Bart the football guy is moving across town
C) One girl got her hair cut and it's way too short.

Pubescent cheerleaders are always in synch, so the answer is likely C. (I of course have no insights in how to find out what the answer *definitely* is, because that would involve your asking a question, which is not safe to do.) But, if the answer *is* C, do not let the ensuing silence throw you once she gets in the car. Simply drive silently yourself, and offer her a tissue. If you *must* say something, say, "There. There." That is all.
DO NOT SAY:

1. "Please stop crying."

How insensitive of you. It's as if there wasn't legitimate reason for her upset.

2. "It must be awful."

How insensitive of you to confirm her suspicions about her horrible hair.

3. "It'll grow back."

How insensitive of you. It's as if you take pleasure in reminding her that it will be a long time before the ordeal is repaired.

4. "I'm sorry."

How insensitive of you. She'll be thinking, "Oh my god I *am* pathetic!"

"There, there" is the safest response. But even that is not without risks.

A cheerleading squad of six, is under the throws of raging hormones every day of the month, and suprisingly, is not always as rational as you might expect.

Walking in on the bridge club

If all eyes turn toward you in stony-cold silence, as if to say you infect their air with your presence…you're fine. You did just interrupt a bridge game, after all. If, however, they're all sampling Helen's upside-down fudge, bundt surprise, and also look at you in stony cold silence, leave for the mall to find a nice gift, taking care to follow the instructions from a couple of paragraphs ago.

Walking in on your wife and her girlfriends having coffee.

If they giggle incessantly when you enter, yes, they were talking about you. If they are terribly angry, it's because you said you were going bowling, and they want some privacy to talk about you. If they say, "Hello" but are actually clenching their teeth, you must turn on your heels and run. Return in three days.

Chapter 10

The Foods We Crave

This chapter is the God's Honest Truth.

At this point, you've undoubtedly put together the food connection. No chapter was complete without touching on it. So, it should come as no surprise when I say to you that at PMS time, we women can be powerful-hungry. Even insatiable. Our desire for fat, salt and sugar can seem highly erratic.

Most women's PMS cravings can be categorized. We tend to fall into one of two groups:
- The salt cravers
- The sweet cravers
(And we're all fat cravers)

These distinctions however, come in a variety of combinations. Consider the PMS cravings combo repertoire:

Salt/Sweet—Most characterized by the need for popcorn and ice cream

Salty/Sour—Often manifests as a desire for potato chips and orange juice

Fatty/Salty—Usually manifested as an overwhelming desire for dozens of bags of anything from Frito-Lay...and French fries.

Fatty/Sweet—Danish pastries and creme' brulee'

I for one, am a fat/sweet craver, predominantly. I can shovel in an entire hot fudge cake in one sitting, and follow it up with a package of cinnamon rolls if I wasn't careful. By careful, I mean, if I didn't bother to follow it up with a box of danish pastries instead. (Anyone knows the Danish pastries include a nutritious fruit filling, and are the healthier choice.)

Many of my friends however, seem to prefer the fatty/salty combo. An entire bag of chips and tub o' dip can be consumed in four and a half seconds.

Let me take a moment to explain.

Why we want more salt.

Our bodies want to die. It is clearly a last minute subconscious attempt to raise our blood pressure and give ourselves a heart attack before bleeding again.

Or: salt makes us swell. Toward kick-off, we want to get it over with. We'd prefer to swell up like a balloon if it would only mean we'd pop sooner.

Why we want more sugar.

We're depressed. We're all swelled up, after all. And how else do you think we get so much manic spurts of cleaning done?

Why we want more fat.

We've got to counter-act the sugar and salt, which are stimulants. Fat slows us down. If we didn't eat it, we'd take over the world, or at least, your tool shed.

If you think your lady's craving for potato chips with onion/cheese dip with an ice cream sandwich chaser is weird, you don't know the half of it.

The following is a list of actually food cravings real people have reported to me. These are truly frightening…all the more so because they are true confessions. That means this is the God's honest truth.

1. Mayonnaise. By the spoon.
2. Creme Brulee and Diet Coke
3. Pepsi chicken. (A recipe that cooks chicken in Pepsi. Swear.)
4. Potato chip-peanut butter sandwiches
5. Sugar sandwiches
6. Raw pancake batter
7. Blood sausage
8. Deep fried fish heads
9. Raw brownies with almond butter
10. The fat trimmings from your steak

Considering the aforementioned, you might take this time to show extra understanding and thoughtfulness towards the lady in your life. Perhaps you can cook for awhile, and experiment with recipes of your own which she might appreciate.

Here, originality counts. Consider a few suggestions.
1. Fruit Loops with fudge sauce
2. Jolly Ranger hard candies dipped in salt.
3. Hebrew National Kosher hot dogs…and butterscotch
4. A salt lick
5. Cocoa puffs with raspberry sauce
6. Pork flavored ice cream
7. Oranges and milk
8. Brownies a la' fried.
9. French Fries and Pina Coladas
10. C&H by the pound

If, you're not creative enough to invent your own meals, I have consolidated a few helpful recipes for you here.

Mud Mountain

(an old family favorite)

Take a mud pie. Stack another on top of it. Cover this with whipped cream, nuts and a cherry. Pour raspberry sauce and Hershey's syrup over the top. Chill. Serves: one.

Mayonaise Pizza

Take a large pepperoni pizza and dollop spoon-sized scoops of Mayo on each piece of Pepperoni. It adds color and is excellent for presentation. Besides, most people will think the mayo is actually goat cheese and will believe you to be a gourmet.

Fudge Tacos (quick and easy)

Purchase some pre-deep fried taco shells at your grocery store. (They keep very well in the cupboard, or frozen for next month.) Open a jar of hot fudge sauce from a quality ice creamery, such as Baskin Robbins. Pour fudge into shell. Heat and serve.

The possibilities are endless. And your lady's love for you will clearly deepen.

Chapter 11

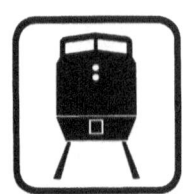

Lead, Follow Or Get Out Of The Way

Okay, gentlemen. It really all boils down to this. The soundest advice I can offer to navigate through this precarious monthly event is, "Lead, Follow, or Get Out Of The Way."

PMS is a time for definitiveness. Conviction. Assertive moves such as running away at a full sprint instead of a jog. Wishy-washy, "helpful" actions will only get you in trouble. Remember, PMS is nothing you can "fix". So, for all you men out there dying to just *make it better*, stop it. Simply go with the flow, (pardon the pun), and let it be. Just be out of the way when the merging of a fan and shit seems inevitable. (When she's shoveling the driveway, and it's July, pick up a shovel and start removing pavement with her. Or, remove yourself.)

Men are From Mars, Women are from Venus, was right. You men have got to support us, let us know we're not crazy when we might appear to be behaving as such. However, that book did not go far enough. Going too far is my job.

WHAT TO DO?

SITUATION:	WISE COURSE OF ACTION:
You go to rent a video.	You keenly recognize this as an ideal time to catch "Ninja Women", "Death Maidens in PJ's", and "Freddy 27", which you've always wanted to see, without argument. These memorable motion pictures you easily snatch from the arms of the other frazzled-looking guy in the action section—he's busy juggling a large bag of french fries in his other hand.
She decides she must clean the closet. Everything in the closet is yours.	With sharply-honed mental reflexes, you announce you Just Need To Be Held for Awhile. Then remind her of your secret fantasy to have something else cleaned and organized in that special way only she can do, say, for example, the sock drawer.
You notice the refrigerator being stocked with something that resembles the contents of the dessert menu at Bubba's House of Ribs & Hot Cakes.	Under the guise of "picking up some potato chips for an appetizer," you step out quickly and get a deli sandwich for dinner. On the way back, you visit your broker and buy stock in Sarah Lee and Hagen Das. You're no dummy. You realize they're going nowhere but up.
She's standing in front of the mirror complaining about bloating.	You throw her on the bed, rip off her clothes and make wild, passionate love to her. (For about 6 1/2 minutes. She has a very short attention span at this point. See chapter 6.)
You catch her openly weeping in response to an infomercial	Run. Run like you've never run before. When you return, bring french fries.
You're in the car and she starts rattling on angrily that you're lost <u>again</u>. And you'll <u>never</u> get to the party!	Distract her with BBQ corn chips. Get the address out of the glove box yourself, then calmly exit your driveway.

In this chapter, I will attempt to further shirk off scientific data, in favor of my own personal experiences, to give you a better understanding of the total female psyche.

I will now attempt to describe the entire PMS phenomenon within a context of the entire female mentality and psychological condition. If, at this point, you're annoyed, believing you could have simply skipped forward to this section, realize please that the other chapters were necessary for the book deal. Otherwise, I would have merely had an "article" deal. Not nearly as financially lucrative. Your reading thus far has not been fruitless.

This is the chapter in which many female psychological mysteries will be revealed. You, the lucky readers of this book, will be enlightened, and the possessors of knowledge so valuable, you could, eventually use it to become a leader of the free world, or at least more competent when ordering dessert at the Olive Garden. But we'll get to that later.

You'll understand more about the entire process, if you first understand the ovaries, and special female idiosyncrasies. Realize first that PMS is a time in which your lady's hormones have found clever new ways to say, "Hey! You're a woman!"

The cycle is a very complex scientific process. It all starts with the ovaries, and let's just begin by saying, the two female ovaries do not get along. They were thrown into each other's company, without so much as an introduction and, as any female will tell you, this is not acceptable for bonding. Unlike males, who need merely a football jersey and a beer to begin spanking each other's behinds affectionately, ("Way to go...uh...what was your name?"), females require common ground, a sense of shared history, and a similar taste in shoes.

So it goes without saying that the two female ovaries spend about 22 days arguing. "*You send the egg.* No...*you* send the egg. *No you!* I did it last time. *No you didn't, I did.* Yeah, and you're so fat you could probably send out four more and not even know the difference!" And so it goes for weeks, until the process exhausts them and one of them finally, "gives it up". In other words, ovulation occurs.

These females are very stubborn. It takes until their late forties for the two of them to finally realize, "Hey! What's all this work about? Why send out eggs anyway?" (Finding a common enemy is the fastest way for females to bond.) "This is really all the *big lady's* fault. We're in the decade of our sexual peak! Let's just make her sweat unexpectedly and grow a mustache. That'll teach the bitch."

Much like the commercials in which gauze-clad, long-haired, flower-holding babes skip in slow motion through a daisy field, into the arms of their adored, after they've consumed unknown quantities of an over-the-counter medication with a flower on the box, your lady will be feeling feminine during this time, but in all the wrong ways. The commercial is a lie.

Being a woman is indeed beautiful. Yet it is full of mysteries...mysteries, which I will unravel for you now. Like peeling away the skin of an onion, I will reveal the many layers of a woman's psyche, and help you understand some of the most vexing of female characteristics. And, much like a peeled onion, they will make your eyes burn until you cry, then leave you wondering if it was worth dealing with the onion in the first place, when garlic works so well.

The 16 Female Mysteries

1. We all have 38 shoes, yet we wear the same two pairs.
Every woman knows that a fashion statement is built from the bottom up. Shoes are the foundation. And some outfits can only be worn with one pair of shoes. Or else we'll die. Therefore, we are mercilessly gripped by an underlying fear that we will be caught, someday, without the right shoes. By "right" we mean, shoes we don't have yet. After all, we're certain there is a photographer from Glamour magazine lying in

wait around every corner attempting to snap our picture and put a black box over our eyes for the fashion "don't" column.

That is why a balanced female psyche requires more shoes than we will ever need. And yes, we wear the black ones with everything. They're comfortable. All the others hurt too much. So we must buy more.

2. We expect you to read our minds.

Of course we do. If you loved us, we wouldn't have to tell you what we wanted. You would just know. The men do in soap operas.

The typical mind-reading expectation goes something like this. You come home from a long day at work. You ask your girlfriend:

You: How are you?
Her: Fine. (angrily)
You: What's wrong?
Her: You don't know?
You: No, I don't.
Her: How could you not know? It's the dishes.
You: I thought you liked them!
Her: How could you get blue! I told you I used to play the French Horn!
You: My insurance is Blue Cross (to the admitting desk of your local mental health facility.)

3. Going to the ladies room in groups

This is for several reasons.

One: we are competitive. We are not about to leave another woman at the table, to be witty, provocative, or change the course of conversation in our absence.

Two: We simply must know what our friend thinks of you so that when we return to the table, we have smirks on our faces and appear to have been giggling incessantly, so as to make our conversation appear harmless, but somehow threatening. It is our birthright to make you nervous, as paybacks for the fact that you didn't call as soon as you said you would on our second date.

Three: It takes awhile. We simply must keep talking.

Four: We have stall doors in our johns. If you didn't have to see *precisely* what it was your buddy was doing before he returned to the table to pass the Dim Sum, you'd go to the john in groups, too.

4. Stuffed animals

We don't really like them. We pretend to so that you will attempt to do something virile for us at carnivals and win more of them with a softball and $10 in quarters. We do this *for you*.

5. Helping each other through *everything*

Helping a girlfriend pick out new pants. Helping a girlfriend decide how to structure the memo. Helping a girlfriend change her hair. We are born "helpers". The truth is, the only people who care what pants to buy, how your hair looks or how the memo reads…are other women. Duh. We constantly seek validation from other women about what other men are thinking, (an undeniably ridiculous approach). This would explain the phenomenon of platform shoes.

6. Ask what you think and then not take the advice.

We do this to confirm our own suspicions that you are usually wrong.

7. The inability to pack light

See mystery #1, above.

8. The inability to move furniture or pack a truck

Woman, on average, are not space-oriented. Unless of course, we're deciding how to make our hair big. The female brain is wired to nurture. To intuit. To *feel*. That is why we can *feel* exactly how heavy the furniture is going to be before we even touch it, and decide to make you do it instead.

9. Talking over every detail of a story 1,000 times

So Ethel got mugged. Every woman knows that what she was wearing, where she was going and why, and the fact that she had just broken up with her boyfriend, and the expression on her face are just as important as that thing the mugger said about a "gun".

10. Not getting to the point

Why should we when what she was wearing, where she was going, and the expression on her face are also so important?

11. The not-expressing-our-opinion phenomenon

Here's the situation. You're in the mall doing some Christmas shopping. You ask your lady, "What would you like for lunch?"

She answers, "Oh, I don't care."

You suggest Chinese.

She says, "Ooh. I don't really feel like Chinese."

You pull out your Blue Cross card again at the same mental health clinic.

The thing is, with other women, we are always at liberty to change our minds. It's what we do. We forget and think we can with you. When you first asked, she *didn't* care. When you suggested Chinese, she did. It's simple really.

12. Demanding caution all the time, then swooning over a reckless Arnold Schwarzennhager character.

You're not Arnold Schwarzennager. He's never had allergies. He doesn't catch cold when he goes out without a sweater. And if one of those bad guys attacks him on the street, he just knocks them out and throws them over his shoulder. You have a bad back.

13. "Am I fat?"
This is also known as the "lose-lose" proposition.

If you say "yes" boy are you in trouble. If you say "no" we call you a liar.

I am telling you now, you want to be a liar. Answer no. Even when we say, "Are you blind?" Even when we say, "Look at this! This is sticking out. I have never been so big." Tell us we are so sexy and thin. Get it? Sexy and we look great. Do not improvise.

You see, the secret is, we *do not want to know if we look fat.* That is *not* what we're asking. Though that may be the words we're using. We want to know if you think we're attractive. Duh. (See mystery #10). And the answer had better damn well be, "You bet!" considering that belly *you've* developed these days.)

15. Dessert—not ordering any but taking quantities of yours
Why order dessert when we know you will? That way, we can pretend we never did. Besides, we just asked you if we look fat.

16. Ask a question and not listen as you answer
Why aren't you following us to make sure we do?

In Conclusion

It's done. That's the conclusion. Come on, I shouldn't have one, you should. Hopefully, it's not divorce. Because you see, we're all like this. But, if you insist on further reading, because you're still as confused as I'm assuming, you might try a few other titles, or, some extra strength Advil. And better luck next month.

About the Author

As an award-winning advertising writer for many years, Kay's written oodles of ads for various national and regional campaigns. Kay's also performed comedy in several clubs and theatres throughout the LA area for quite awhile too. But her greatest talent is writing glowing things about herself in bios.

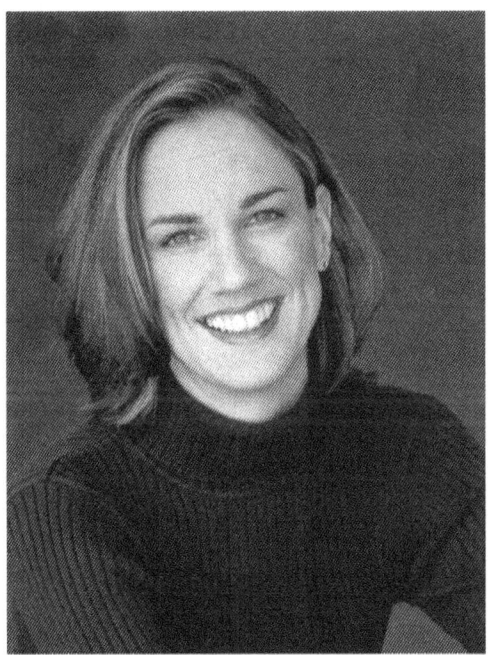

Appendix I

Suggested Readings
    The Taming of The Shrew, William Shakespeare
    Mating Rituals in the Lower Atarondacks
    Dr. Seuss. (Any title)
    My Life As A Female Wrestler
    Paul Perdue's Southern Fried Cooking
    Women Who Feel Like The Wolves
    Chicken Soup is for the soul. (Not the book. Read the label. There's lots' of fat in each can.)

Suggested Book Burnings:
    Our Bodies, Ourselves
    The Blue Lagoon. Nuf said.
    The Victoria's Secret Catalog…the one piece of literature both sexes usually love. (Don't worry. They send out plenty. You'll have another in four days.)

Appendix II

Ten Suggested Activities and Future Projects to make the most of PMS

1. The building of that Mexico/U.S. wall Pat kept going on about.
2. Cleaning the lint from the slats in your hairdryer
3. Moving
4. The annexation of Cuba
5. Moving Cuba further away
6. Watching "Gone With The Wind" repeatedly until you learn all the dialogue (see Chapter 8)
7. Wind sprints
8. Scouring the hull of the Queen Mary in dry dock.
9. The "New" Betty Crocker Bake-Off
10. The Ultimate Fighting Challenge. For women.

Appendix III

Men's 10 Biggest PMS Mistakes and How to Avoid Them
Well, Sherlock, that's what the whole book was about. But, consider this part a handy reference, or concordance, like in the back of the bible, to look up where you may need extra review.

1. Trying to fix it.
See chapters 1, 3, 5 and 8.

2. Assuming it will last forever.
See chapter 2. Wait for half-time.

3. Not recognizing it.
See chapter 1.

4. Enlisting your mate's assistance in *your* agenda.
See chapters 7 and 8.

5. Making Love.
At this time, you're *having sex*. See chapter 5.

6. Spooning.
It reminds her of food. See chapter 10.

7. Asking if it's *that time*.
Whoa. Don't ever ask! See chapter 1.

8. Taking a vacation.
Better to send her on one. See chapters 1 and 8.

9. Starting a diet.
See chapter 10.

10. Breathing.
This is somewhat difficult to avoid. However, you should try. After all, any of your annoying eccentricities can be especially vexing during this sensitive time. Even if it is simply your existence.

Appendix IV

A Couple's Exercise

Here is your chance to prove to your lady that you do understand. That you've read up on the subject. That you're a kindred spirit.

Give her this list, or better still, do this exercise together, and you'll get some tonight. (And don't spaz. You know they send you multiple copies of that thing. Just keep *yours*).

12 Creative Ways to Destroy the Victoria's Secret Catalogue

1. Scotch tape it to your bumper and enter the 405 freeway.

2. Unfold it to her favorite model, tie the catalogue to a stake, and burn them for witchcraft.

3. Throw it into the washing machine. Add bleach.

4. Make origami birds out of various pages. Then scatter the birdies around your driveway. And drive.

5. Ask your nephew for his Mr. Wizard chemistry set. Give anyone she chooses a nasty skin disease.

6. Get a puppy. Line his dog house with it.

7. Learn to scuba dive. Feed the sharks.

8. Go to the Hollywood Christmas parade. She'll need something to protect her feet from the gutter.

9. Walk the puppy you just bought, and pick up his doodies with it.

10. Make a ransom note out of its clippings…to teach the other catalogues a lesson

11. Put it on the paper towel rack in your kitchen. Rip off separate pages to mop up spills. Like, spills of broccoli soup.

12. Have her send clippings of it with clever notes in the margin…to her ex-boyfriends', girlfriends' houses.